Belly Fat
Conspiracies

Four Theories About

What Is Behind The

Belly Fat Epidemic

K. L. Becker

First Printing, 2013

ISBN-13: 978-1492124832
ISBN-10: 1492124834

Printed in the United States of America

Disclaimer

This publication is designed to provide accurate and authoritative information in regard to the subject matter covered. It is sold with the understanding that the publisher is not engaged in rendering health, legal, nutritional, accounting, or other professional services. If professional advice or other expert assistance is required, the services of a competent professional person should be sought. Designated trademarks and brands are the property of their respective owners.

CONTENTS

INTRODUCTION

What's Up With That Fat Belly?

Belly Fat seems to be the current fashionable "moniker" for today. The popular nametags for this condition in the past are: a beer belly, a spare tire, having a pear shape, the middle age spread or your love handles. Medical professionals such as physicians and nurses often refer to this condition as abdominal obesity. I'll keep up with the current trend and refer to it as fat belly.

Does it seem to you that there is an unusually high pitch about fat bellies these days? In fashion are cures for fat bellies, guidebooks for belly fat, cookbooks for belly fat, and exercises for belly fat…on and on. Not only is there quite a bit of fervor about this subject among the public but there have been some highly credentialed professionals that have made belly fat there "mission" and there has been some highly respected institutions that have conducted research on this subject.

What Is Behind This Phenomenon?

Well I'm sure it is not a surprise to you that we are experiencing an obesity epidemic in much of the developed world. We are fatter than ever and getting fatter every day. Belly fat is "popping up or more accurately flopping over" more and more every day. It seems to me that it's not just a fat belly problem it is a problem with fat thighs, fat buttocks, fat arms and fat necks. Pretty much every body part where you can "pinch a handful of fat" is the problem. Using the proper medical terminology let's call it the subcutaneous fat (fat under the skin) problem.

It's just that when we look in a full length mirror, we "pull up our trousers" or strap on the seatbelt, our belly fat is the first thing that comes to our attention…over and over. Fat bellies are very unsightly and very uncomfortable. Constantly dealing with belly fat can lead to declining self-confidence as our self-image deteriorates. Not to mention what a toll on our daily energy the belly fat takes. Soon we begin to notice how getting up the stairs or walking even short distances becomes increasingly more difficult.

Are There Unseen Forces Conspiring To Expand Your Waste Line?

Many of us are struggling to cinch up our belts to the "notch of years ago" but are just not making the progress we would like to. Cutting back on favorite desserts, resisting second helpings, drinking fewer beers, untold stomach crunches…nothing works. So you go online and search for help.

What you find might surprise you. Belly Fat Conspiracies: Powerful forces at work keeping your waist in an ever increasing state. Who are they and what do they have to gain from doing this? If there are fat belly conspiracies, who cares anyway? What's the problem with carrying this pouch around? So many of us carry one now days.

1 BELLY FAT IS NOT JUST UNSIGHTLY

There is a problem with belly fat that other fat body parts don't have in common. That is when someone has belly fat they also are at a rather high risk of having what is commonly called in the medical industry as fatty liver. And possibly even extra fat layering around their heart. This visceral fat is far more serious to a person's health than if appearance were the only issue. Visceral fat layered within the abdomen more easily breaks down into fatty acids than other types of fat. This fatty acid ends up getting deposited directly into the liver thus eventually causing the fatty liver syndrome.

Alcohol Is Particularly Concerning

If alcohol is to blame for belly fat then most probably the liver is also fat. Large alcohol consumers are at a very high risk of having a fatty liver. In fact, more than eighty percent of people who abuse alcohol develop chronic fatty liver disease often referred to as cirrhosis of the liver a condition where the liver enlarges and, slowly over time, normal functioning liver cells are replaced with scar tissue. This disease often leads to liver dysfunction, liver failure and ultimately death. So if your belly fat is caused by too much alcohol consumption get on a plan to substantially reduce the alcohol you are drinking or better yet stop drinking it all together as soon as possible.

Even Non-Drinker Belly Fat Has Risk

Nonalcoholic fatty livers may not lead to serious health problems if the condition does not trigger inflammation or damage to the liver as described above. However, fatty livers not caused by alcohol are present in nearly twenty percent of adults and can also lead to cirrhosis and other serious liver conditions. Obese children can be subjected to this malady and if so are at a much higher than normal risk of developing heart disease as well.

Researching the health problems associated with a fat belly will uncover many more maladies that health professionals, researchers and health publishers attribute to it. Another serious health problem attributed to belly fat is heart disease. Not only can visceral fat engulf your liver and kill you it can also shroud your heart causing it to work harder than it should to pump blood throughout your body.

Visceral fat (fat located deep in your body around organs not right under the skin) has been found to cause inflammation by breaking down into hormones in the blood stream that inflame the tissue your internal organs are made of. As you may already know, inflammation is a major risk factor for heart disease as it contributes to hardening of the arteries. So your heart is laboring to pump blood because of the fat surrounding it AND the arteries it is trying to pump the blood through are getting narrower and narrower eventually leading to a heart attack.

More Health Risks Associated With Abdominal Obesity

With some of these health conditions there is not an obvious connection to fat bellies that makes sense logically to the non-health professional, but here they are:

High cholesterol and triglycerides
High blood pressure
Stroke
Insulin resistance and diabetes
Erectile dysfunction
Kidney, breast, uterine, cervix, colon and pancreas cancer

So all of these health risks should give everyone motivation to jump on the current "belly fat" bandwagon and figure out what to do about it.

2 CONSPIRACY THEORY #1

On the surface of it you would think that it would be real easy to figure out what causes belly fat: Eating and drinking way too much of the wrong things! Seems pretty simple…right? Well dig into it a little deeper and you will uncover a few conspiracy theories! Some out there are selling the idea that it's really not your fault that you have belly fat. There are sinister forces at work conspiring to add more and more inches to your waist line every year. And, without the help of those who have uncovered these conspiracies you will be helpless to do anything about it.

Conspiracy Theory Number One – It's Sugar

Yep, your waist line is ever expanding because mankind invented refined sugar and man-made refined sugar is now added to nearly everything we eat in such huge quantities that there is no way for our bodies to handle all of the sugar with normal dieting and accepted run of the mill weight loss programs.

Sugar-Aholics

Upon investigating this I conjure up visions of food companies processing the fiber out of most of the food we purchase and adding in loads of sugar, not to speak of fat and salt, to make their food taste as good as possible so that we will become "processed food addicts" craving sugar highs and needing more and more of them everyday.

To The Rescue

Not to worry! Throw away everything you have learned about "calories in and calories out" dieting and get on this special sugar-free diet to get your sugar consumption down to what it was when pre-historic man consumed sugar only from natural foods and natural food sugar was hard to come by because there were no pre-historic supermarkets to go to. Sugar is what triggers insulin and insulin carries the sugar (glucose) right into your cells to be burned for energy or stored as fat. Fat and protein are not the culprits.

In fact, this "sugar revelation" is so revolutionary that you don't need to worry about counting calories, or giving up the foods you love. It's OK to eat bacon, sausage, hamburgers and, of course, T-bones. Just minimize all sugar and processed carbohydrates and you are going to drop the belly fat like no other diet or weight loss system you have ever tried within a week or two.

No Need To Exercise?

And guess what else? You don't even have to worry about exercise! It's all in controlling your blood sugar and insulin. Stay away from ALL sugar even what's in fresh fruit and especially sugary beverages like…skim milk. Don't worry about fat-free. Fat is not a problem because it does not contain any sugar.

Some In The Weight Loss (Belly Fat) Community Are Not Buying

Needless to say, many nutritionists are not jumping on the sugar-free only diet. Most agree that there is certainly too much sugar in everyone's diet and controlling sugar consumption is absolutely warranted but they object to not tracking or even paying attention to other nutrients such as trans or saturated fat, salt, fiber, vitamins or even calories.

3 CONSPIRACY THEORY #2

Conspiracy Theory Number Two – It's Wheat

Here is another popular theory. Your belly fat is not caused by your overeating high calorie fattening food; it is really caused by the wheat you are eating. This sounds a little like the sugar conspiracy because the root of the problem comes from man made, or more accurately, man engineered wheat. You see for the past several decades the agricultural industry has been cross breeding and perhaps even genetically engineering the wheat they plant in their fields to maximize the yield and minimize the cost of growing their wheat.

Super Bad Wheat

The idea is that if they can grow wheat that becomes less and less thirsty for water and more and more resistant to insects thus requiring less pesticides, the more profitable and richer they will get. And, it seems they certainly have been successful in increasing the yield per acre planted throughout the years. This begs the question: How well does the human body process this super-wheat? The wheat conspiracy alleges that the strains of wheat we are eating today are wreaking havoc with our digestive system's capability to process it into the energy we intend to get when eating it.

Whole Grains Are Bad?

Now here is the really bad part according to the super bad wheat theorists: Most of the time when we seek professional advice about weight loss and dieting we are told that the problem is we are eating too much fattening food that we need to cut back on and replace it with guess what?...whole grains! Just the opposite of what we should do to "kick the wheat addiction." The entire calorie counting and calorie-in calorie-out dieting industry that has been around for years and years is wrong and is now out. No need to count calories or worry about fat in your diet. Also, your belly fat is not really about how much exercise you do either.

We Were Made To Be Meat Eaters Not Wheat Eaters

The theory goes that the human species was not "made" originally to eat grains for sustenance. We were created as carnivores or meat eaters, if you like, and we did not start eating grain until about ten thousand years ago. This mistake today is compounded by not only the agricultural business "frankensteining" our wheat but now wheat is in almost every last thing we put in our mouths...even soup and the dressing we put on salad. Are the farmers and food companies "conspiring" to put this engineered freak wheat in everything we eat because they know it will create binge eating and food addictions? Kind of sounds like a drug cartel...doesn't it? Let's call it the freak wheat cartel.

The Amazing Affects of Breaking Free of Freak Wheat

Amazingly, there are stories about when victims of the freak wheat cartel finally are able to be "gluten clean" age old health problems that they have been dealing with for most of their lives vanish. Some claim to lose up to forty pounds in as little as three months. Aches and pains go away.

Asthma and arthritis symptoms are either reduced or gone for good for some wheat-free eaters. Others claim that irritable bowl conditions are cured and blood sugar comes back into balance. It has been reported that when super bad freak wheat is eliminated from their diet, maladies such as hypertension and acid reflux are dealt with.

It's Highly Addictive

Super-bad freak wheat first of all creates uncontrollable so called "carb cravings" that lead to binge overeating and obesity. As we know already obesity leads to blood sugar imbalances and diabetes. So, even diabetes is reported to be controlled with a wheat free diet.

Wheat "Allergy" And Celiac Disease

There is a well know condition that many people have called celiac disease which is a lack of a person's ability to properly digest gluten proteins found in wheat and other grains. This can be a serious disease with sometimes debilitating digestive track symptoms such as chronic constipation or diarrhea among others. Additionally, some people have a simple allergy to gluten. In both instances life-long gluten free diets will result in vast improvements in, not only digestive disorders, but a patient's overall health.

It would seem according to the super bad freak wheat theorists we all have some kind of mutant gluten disorder that "feeds" on itself. Thinking about this freak wheat belly fat theory brings one thing to mind: If our wheat now is over hybridized and genetically engineered to create a super "Frankenstein" wheat drug like food staple, what about all of the antibiotics and "bred to be fat animals" we are eating. Do we have Frankenstein meat on our plate too?

4 CONSPIRACY THEORY #3

Conspiracy Theory Number Three
You Aren't Getting Enough Vitamin D

Here is how this theory goes. Supposedly a study focusing on bone mass in women uncovered some unexpected results: A correlation between low levels of vitamin D and unusually high "pinch able" amounts of abdominal fat. In fact, it was reported that in women a vitamin D deficiency (less than 20ng/ml) group had 80% more belly fat than women with adequate vitamin D in their blood stream. It was reported that older ages had a higher negative correlation than younger aged women.

It turns out that a person's kidneys will transform Vitamin D into a hormone called 1,25-D that your body utilizes to control the growth of cells in your body, including fat cells. So if you have enough of this hormone in your bloodstream fat cells will actually shrink or "drain". Also an adequate amount of Vitamin D helps your liver break down fat cells more efficiently and it will even reduce a person's appetite along with increasing muscle. Anybody interested in buying Vitamin D Supplements?

5 CONSPIRACY THEORY #4

Conspiracy Theory Number Four – Dieting

Yes, you read this right. There is a well known doctor that has a show and is interviewed quite frequently regarding healthy living. The theory he touts goes like this: Dieting is very stressful and it is a well known fact that stress is a major contributor to adding fat not only to bellies but everywhere. Stress releases a hormone called cortisol. Cortosil is the hormone your body uses to help you when there is something in your environment that threatens you. Cortosil and Adrenalin are the main hormones responsible in your body to prepare you to fight or run (flight) when you become frightened or angry at something you have encountered.

The Fight or Flight Response

As soon as you hear gun shots, screeching tires, smell smoke or whatever the perceived threat is the hypothalamus at the base of your brain triggers alarms by firing off certain nerves. When the adrenal glands located near your kidneys detect the alarm they start dumping cortosil and adrenalin into your bloodstream. The adrenalin causes your heart to start beating faster thus increasing your blood pressure.

Preparing Your Body For The State You Are In

This bodily response is for the purposes of supplying your muscle cells with more energy. Cortosil is the hormone that helps boost the energy carried to your cells by increasing the sugar in your bloodstream called glucose. It also performs work on other functions in your body to make you into the best fighting or fight machine you are capable of being.

Cortosil will help your brain to process glucose more efficiently allowing you to be alert and thinking clearly. It will increase the material in your bloodstream that your body uses to repair damaged tissue in case you are injured. It also enhances your immune system to fight infections that you might get from this threat and it slows down your digestive, reproduction and growth systems in your body to conserve whatever energy they may be taking.

When Your Body Thinks The Threat Never Goes Away

So you should be grateful your body secretes such a high powered hormone when you need it. However, when you are constantly under stress and the fight or flight reaction is not temporary, your body never gets back to its normal state. Your heart rate and blood pressure remain constantly high caused by your body always being alarmed and it reacts as if it is faced with constant threats.

All of the body functions never achieve normal relaxed states, including the glucose in your bloodstream. If you don't burn off this extra glucose it goes right into storage...more and more fat...especially in the belly. Also, while dieting you are constantly hungry and the hunger is made worse by your body thinking it needs more stored energy to respond to the "famine".

So if you are obsessing over every calorie and worrying about every bite you eat, so the theory goes, dieting will actually have the opposite effect you are looking to achieve. Your body will try and "fight or flight from" your diet.

6 WHAT YOU CAN DO TO FIGHT BACK

I would recommend that the very first thing you can do is view every product that is being pitched to you with claims that someone behind the product has discovered a "secret key", a one overriding factor, that if you buy into their theory and buy their products your belly fat will magically disappear without having to count calories, worry about exercise or stop eating fattening foods with a very skeptical attitude.

Some of the conspiracy theorists do have highly respected credentials…like MD. However, I have done business in my lifetime with MD's that, at the end of the day, it was obvious their pocketbook was a higher priority than my health.

Who Knows…All Of These Fat Belly Theories Could Be Right

It is not my purpose to refute or disparage ANY of these belly fat theories. I do not have the scientific evidence to do so. There are many testimonials that claim wondrous results when buying and using the solutions and products sold by the belly fat theorists. However, there also are many negative testimonials that cry about no results.

You have to make up your own mind. I would recommend that you base your opinion on sound scientific evidence conducted by independent well respected medical institutions that have conducted statistically significant studies not only for the belly fat theory you are investigating but also have a track record of completing studies similar to the one used as proof that the fat belly theorist's claims are "scientifically valid".

CONCLUSION

Maybe Belly Fat Is Our Fault

In thinking about all of these belly fat theories, a self help meeting I attended in the past comes to mind. I remember vividly the speaker standing in front of the audience then making everyone stand up and repeat "I AM RESPOMSIBLE". My opinion is that some of this thinking is appropriate with these belly fat causes and solutions. How is it possible to lose belly fat when the belly fat owner ingests way more food (calories) than they burn off every day? If they cut out sugar or wheat or load up on vitamin D but still have a very large calorie surplus, are they really going to lose belly fat?

Lastly, if they don't count the calories they eat and burn everyday (keep score) will they even know whether they have a calorie deficient or surplus every day, every week, every year?

Ask yourself these questions and then ask yourself this question: Is there really a sinister conspiracy adding inches to your belt or should you just make some not too difficult and not too expensive life-style changes involving what you eat and how you exercise? A change that will result in weight loss of one to two pounds per week. A change that will not result in constant hunger and will be easy to maintain over the long haul.

ABOUT THE AUTHOR

K. L. Becker is dedicated to providing useful information regarding weight loss, fat reduction, exercise and other healthy life-style choices. Please visit:

www.weightlossextrabonus.com/beckerbooks

You Will find more useful publications related to fat and weight loss and calorie counting.

Thanks For Purchasing This Book

As a special thanks for purchasing this book I am going to give you a special bonus report on nutrition. Please go to:

www.weightlossextrabonus.com